THE BODY RESET

Revamp Your Health in Just 3 Weeks
with Simple, Science-Backed
Strategies

PHARM. CHARITY O.

Dedication

This great and mindset-transforming book is dedicated to everyone who will employ the simple, science-backed strategies in this book to revamp their health in just 3 weeks.

Table of Contents

Hello, and thank you for choosing to check out "The Body Reset: Revamp Your Health in Just 3 Weeks with Simple, Science-Backed Strategies"! Are you sick of how sluggish, overweight, and unfit makes you feel? Are you sick of trendy diets that promise instant results but never deliver anything worthwhile? If that's the case, you should read this book.

You'll find a powerful and actionable plan for altering your health in just three weeks within the following pages of this document. This book is not a diet; rather, it is a reset of your system. You will learn how to restore your health and vitality by fueling your body with complete, healthy foods, boosting your energy and metabolism, and reclaiming your health and vitality if you follow the straightforward tactics that are given in this article.

"The Body Reset" can help you achieve your goals, whether they are to reduce body fat, increase your level of physical fitness, or feel better overall. We will discuss the research that underpins the program and then walks you through the process of incorporating it into your day-to-day life step by step. When you've finished reading this book, you'll have the information and resources you need to make changes to your body and life that are both healthy and long-lasting.

This program's straightforwardness is one reason for its resounding success. We have eliminated all of the unnecessary features and tricks to zero down on effective ones. You won't find any elaborate meal planning or stringent guidelines to adhere to in this guide. Instead, you will acquire the knowledge necessary to make dietary decisions that are beneficial to both your body and your way of life in a healthy and nourishing way.

You'll also learn why it's so important to get some form of physical activity into your daily routine, and how even a modest quantity of physical activity may significantly influence your overall health and sense of well-being. We will provide you with strategies and methods for incorporating physical activity into your hectic schedule, as well as assistance in locating activities that spark your interest.

Yet "The Body Reset" isn't only about changing your diet and doing more exercise. When it comes to your health, it's important to take a holistic approach and make sure you're addressing all of the aspects that play a role in your well-being.

This is the reason why we have included chapters on how to manage stress, how to get enough sleep, and how to change your perspective. You will be able to build a solid base for yourself that will serve as a pillar in all aspects of your life if you pay attention to these critical aspects.

So, if you are prepared to move toward a better and happier version of yourself, let's begin with this guide!

Chapter 1

WHAT THE BODY RESET IS AND WHY YOU SHOULD CONSIDER DOING IT.

Hello, and welcome to the Body Reset program! Throughout the next three weeks, you will get started on a path to improve your health and well-being using straightforward methods that are supported by scientific research.

But before we get into that, let's discuss what the Body Reset is and how it might be of use to you.

This approach is not a diet in any way. It is a holistic approach to health and wellness that focuses on fueling your body with full, nourishing meals, boosting your energy and metabolism with physical exercise, and developing a healthy foundation by managing stress, getting enough sleep, and maintaining a positive mentality.

In contrast to many other diets that promise instant results, the Body Reset is intended to be followed for the long term and may be tailored to your requirements and tastes. It's about making changes to your body and your life that are good for you and that last.

Thus, why should you consider the body Reset? Only a handful of the reasons are as follows:

It's not hard at all. We have eliminated all of the unnecessary features and tricks to zero down on those that are effective. You won't find any elaborate meal planning or stringent guidelines to adhere to in this guide.

It is based on scientific evidence. The approaches that are discussed in this book are derived from the most recent findings of research and suggestions made by specialists in the domains of nutrition, physical activity, and overall wellness.

It can be adapted to your needs. You will acquire the knowledge necessary to make decisions that are beneficial to both your body and your way of life, as well as the skills necessary to incorporate regular physical activity into your routine.

The approach is holistic. If you pay attention to every facet of your health and well-being, you'll be able to establish a solid base that will serve as a pillar for you in every facet of your life.

The Body Reset is perfect for you if you are prepared to take charge of your health and begin feeling like the finest version of yourself. Let's get started!

The Body Reset program's ease of use is one reason for its widespread popularity. We have made the program simple to understand and implement, using tactics that are lucid and uncomplicated, and which can readily be included in your day-to-day activities.

You will devote the first week of the program to focusing on providing your body with whole meals that are beneficial to its health. This involves opting for meals that have been processed to a minimum, have a high nutrient content, and are enjoyable to consume. You will learn how to read food labels, how to make better choices while shopping for groceries and dining out, and how to increase the proportion of your diet that consists of fruits, vegetables, and other whole foods.

You will also gain an understanding of the function that carbs, proteins, and fats play in your diet, as well as the proper way to balance these macronutrients to achieve optimum health. You will learn about the advantages of fiber and how to incorporate an adequate amount of fiber into your diet. You will also understand the significance of hydration and the best practices for maintaining adequate hydration throughout the day.

Yet, the Body Reset is not only concerned with one's diet. You'll also gain an understanding of how physical activity can increase your level of energy as well as your metabolism and overall well-being. We will provide you with helpful hints and strategies for squeezing physical activity into your hectic schedule, as well as suggestions for activities that you find enjoyable. You'll learn about the advantages of strength training, cardiovascular exercise, and flexibility training and how to include all three in your regimen.

At the end of the first week, you will have a strong basis upon which to develop a nutritious, nourishing diet and an active lifestyle. You'll be well on your way to accomplishing your health and wellness goals as well as feeling as good as you possibly can.

So, let's get started!

Chapter 2

WEEK 1: FOCUSES ON PROVIDING YOUR BODY WITH WHOLE FOODS THAT ARE NOURISHING TO IT.

Hello, and welcome to the first week of the Body Reset! This week, you will concentrate on providing your body with whole foods that are beneficial to its health. This involves opting for meals that have been processed to a minimum, have a high nutrient content, and are enjoyable to consume.

But why is it so necessary to emphasize foods that are both whole and nourishing? Only a handful of the causes are as follows:

Whole foods are typically considered to have the highest nutrient density. They are packed with a wide array of vitamins, minerals, and other critical micronutrients that your body needs to function at its absolute best. You can ensure that you are getting all of the nutrients your body and mind require if you choose a wide variety of whole foods to eat. This will support both your body and your mind.

Consuming foods that are both whole and nourishing will assist you in feeling fuller and content. The high fiber content of many whole foods contributes to the satiety and fullness that can be achieved after eating them. This may be of particular use to you if you are attempting to reduce your body fat percentage or keep it at a healthy level.

Consuming foods that are both whole and nourishing can help one maintain a healthy weight. When it comes to weight management, the quantity of calories you consume is one of the most important factors. However, the quality of the calories you consume is also very important. Whole, wholesome foods are typically better for managing one's weight because they contain fewer calories and more nutrients per serving than processed foods.

The question now is how you may improve your diet to include more whole foods that are rich in nutrients. Try your hand at some of these different strategies:

Create a list of the things that you need to buy. Make a list of the whole, wholesome foods that you want to buy before going to the grocery store and stick to the list.

You'll be better able to maintain your focus and resist the need to make impulsive purchases as a result.

Select foods that are whole and not processed. Choose foods that are whole, unprocessed, and unpackaged wherever feasible instead of ones that have been excessively processed or packaged.

Try out a variety of different dishes. You should make it a weekly goal to include at least one new fruit or vegetable in your diet. This will not only assist you in obtaining a greater range of nutrients, but it also has the potential to make your meals more interesting and pleasurable to eat.

If you follow these tactics, you will be well on your way to sustaining your body with meals that are entire and nourishing when you eat them. In the following chapter, we will discuss ways in which you can increase both your energy and your metabolism through physical activity.

In addition to selecting foods that are complete and nutrient-dense, it is essential to give careful **consideration to the proportions of the macronutrients (carbohydrates, proteins, and fats) that make up your diet.** Because of the varied functions that each macronutrient performs in the body, striking the appropriate dietary balance is critical to achieving and maintaining optimum health.

The following is a concise explanation of the function served by each macronutrient:

Carbohydrates: Carbohydrates are the primary source of energy that is used by your body. They can be found in a wide range of foods, such as fruits, vegetables, grains, and legumes, among other things. It is essential to select complex carbohydrates, which include foods like legumes and whole grains because of their high content of fiber and minerals. Steer clear of refined carbohydrates like white bread and sugary snacks if you want to avoid gaining weight. These foods are low in nutrients and contribute to weight gain.

Proteins: Proteins are essential for the development and repair of tissues, as well as the preservation of healthy muscles, bones, and skin. Both animal and plant sources include them; examples of the former include meat, chicken, fish, eggs, and dairy products, while examples of the latter include beans, nuts, and seeds. Make it a goal to receive protein from a wide variety of sources in your diet.

Fats: Fats are an important source of energy, and they also assist your body in absorbing certain nutrients. Fats help your body absorb certain nutrients. On the other hand, it is essential to select good fats, such as monounsaturated and polyunsaturated fats, which are present in foods such as olive oil, avocados, almonds, and seeds, among other places. Avoid eating fried foods and processed snacks because they contain unhealthy fats like trans and saturated fats. These fats can be found in fried foods.

You can provide for the energy requirements of your body and improve your overall health by paying attention to the balance of the macronutrients in your food.

Consuming an adequate amount of fiber is another essential component of providing adequate nourishment to your body. Your body is unable to digest the type of carbohydrate known as fiber, but this does not negate the fact that fiber is beneficial to your overall health. It helps you feel full and pleased throughout the day, and it also has the potential to reduce the risk of heart disease and other health concerns. Whole grains, fruits, vegetables, and legumes are all excellent food choices that are high in fiber. Try to consume between 25 and 30 grams of fiber every single day.

In conclusion, it is essential to maintain proper hydration throughout the day by consuming enough amount of fluids at regular intervals. The ideal option is water, but you can also acquire fluids from other sources, such as fruits, vegetables, and soups made with broth. Strive to consume at least 8 cups, which is equal to 64 ounces, of fluids daily.

If you follow these principles, you will be well on your way to fueling your body with entire meals that are beneficial to your health. In the following chapter, we will discuss ways in which you can increase both your energy and your metabolism through physical activity.

Chapter 3

WEEK 2: INCREASE YOUR ENERGY LEVELS AND IMPROVE YOUR METABOLISM THROUGH WORKOUT AND MOVEMENT

Hello, and welcome to the second week of the Body Reset! This week, you will concentrate on improving your energy levels and metabolism through increased movement and exercise.

But why exactly is it so crucial that you work some form of physical activity into your daily schedule? Only a handful of the advantages are as follows:

The metabolic rate can be increased through physical activity. When you exercise, the calories stored in your body are burned off and used as fuel for your activities. This has the potential to assist you in boosting your resting metabolism, which refers to the number of calories that your body burns while it is at rest.

Your cardiovascular health can be improved with the use of exercise. The chance of developing heart disease can be lowered, your cholesterol levels can be improved, and your blood pressure can be lowered when you engage in regular physical activity.

Exercising regularly can give you more energy. Even though it might not make sense at first glance, physical activity can boost your energy levels. Endorphins are chemicals that are produced in your body when you engage in physical activity. These chemicals can help to improve your mood and boost your energy levels.

Physical activity has been shown to promote mental wellness. It has been demonstrated that participating in regular physical activity can boost mood, lower stress levels, and overall increase mental well-being.

Thus, what are some ways that you may include more physical activity and exercise into your daily routine? **Try your hand at some of these different strategies:**

Find activities you enjoy. Picking out physical activities that you take pleasure in doing is essential if you want to maintain an exercise routine. This could be anything from walking, running, or cycling to yoga, dancing, or swimming. Other possibilities include all of these things. Discovering activities that you look forward to participating in is the most significant step to take.

Develop it into a routine. If you want to make physical activity a consistent part of your life, you should strive to exercise at the same time every day. This might take place right when you get up in the morning, over your lunch break, or after you clock out for the day.

Start small. Begin slowly and steadily increasing the intensity of your workout if you are new to working out or if it has been a long since you have been physically active. To reap the benefits of exercise, it is not necessary to perform strenuous workouts daily. A difference can be made with as little as a few minutes of effort.

If you follow these tips, you'll be well on your way to improving your energy levels and metabolism through movement and exercise. In the following chapter, we will concentrate on developing a healthy foundation by learning how to manage stress, getting enough sleep, and changing our perspective.

In addition to selecting physical activities that you enjoy doing, it is essential to mix up your training routine to present your body with a variety of new challenges. This can help to keep your workouts interesting and avoid you from becoming bored while you're doing them.

There are primarily three categories of physical activity: cardio, strength training, and flexibility training. The following is a concise explanation of each:

Cardiovascular exercise: Any activity that gets your heart rate up and keeps it there for a sustained period is considered to be cardiovascular exercise. Cardiovascular exercise, also known as cardio, is another name for this type of exercise. Activities such as strolling, jogging, cycling, swimming, and dancing are examples. You may improve your cardiovascular health, raise your metabolism, and improve your endurance by participating in cardiovascular exercise. Strive to do at least 150 minutes of cardiovascular activity per week at a moderate intensity or 75 minutes of cardiovascular activity at a strong intensity.

Strength training: The term "strength training" refers to any physical exercise in which your muscles are challenged by the application of resistance. Weights, resistance bands, or even just your body weight can be used to accomplish this. The accumulation of muscle mass, as well as bone density and metabolic rate, can be improved with resistance exercise. Try to perform some form of resistance training at least twice a week, focusing on all of the major muscle groups.

The range of motion that can be achieved in a person's joints is referred to as flexibility. Yoga and stretching are two practices that can assist in the development of greater flexibility. Increased flexibility can aid in the correction of poor posture, lessen the strain placed on muscles, and lessen the likelihood of injury. Your goal should be to perform flexibility exercises at least twice a week.

You can put your body through a variety of different kinds of challenges and develop a well-rounded fitness program by including a wide range of different types of physical activities in your routine.

It is also essential that you pay attention to the requirements of your body and pay attention to how it feels. It is acceptable to reduce the intensity of your workouts or take a break if you are experiencing muscle soreness or fatigue. The most important thing is to find a good equilibrium that suits your needs.

If you follow these instructions, you will be well on your way to increase both your energy level and your metabolism through exercise and movement. In the following chapter, we will concentrate on developing a healthy foundation by learning how to manage stress, getting enough sleep, and changing our perspective.

It is essential to take into consideration not only the positive effects that exercise has on one's body, but also the positive effects that it has on one's mind. Exercising has been demonstrated to have a positive effect on mood, lower stress levels, and improve general mental health.

Listed below are a few of the many ways that physical activity can improve your mental health:

Exercising can be an effective way to alleviate tension and anxiety. Endorphins are naturally occurring chemicals that are produced in the body as a result of physical activity. Endorphins have been shown to improve mood and lower levels of stress. A sense of accomplishment and a diversion from negative thoughts are two additional benefits that come with regular physical activity.

Workouts can improve sleep. It has been shown that engaging in regular physical activity can improve the quality of sleep that one receives and the quantity of time spent in deep sleep. You may wake up feeling revitalized and ready to take on the day if you do this before bed.

Exercise can increase self-esteem. Seeing positive changes in your body as a result of your exercise routine may be a great confidence and esteem booster. Doing regular exercise can also make you feel like you have a better handle on both your life and your body.

You may enhance your physical and emotional well-being by making exercise a regular part of your routine and reaping the benefits of doing so.

In addition to this, it is essential to develop strategies to make physical activity joyful. This can make it easier for you to stay motivated and increase your likelihood of continuing your fitness routine. **Try your hand at some of these ideas:**

Do your workouts with a buddy or a member of the family. Having a workout partner can assist in making your workouts more fun, as well as give encouragement and support.

Experiment with a new activity. Switch to something else whenever you get bored with the task you were doing before.

Try going to a different place. Altering the setting where you complete your workouts helps keep things interesting and presents fresh challenges. This could entail exercising in the great outdoors, at a local park, or even at a gym.

Discover a way to exercise that complements your unique character. Are you a social person? Think about signing up for a team sport or a fitness class with other people. Do you like alone activities? Try running, cycling, or yoga. Increase the likelihood that you will like your exercises by picking activities that are a good fit for your character and interests.

Reward yourself. Rewarding oneself after achieving a fitness goal is a good approach to keep yourself motivated to continue working out. This could be something trivial, such as a nutritious snack or a massage, or it could be something more substantial, such as a new piece of exercise equipment or a vacation. Make sure to pick out incentives that contribute to your efforts to improve your general health and well-being.

Make exercise a part of your routine that you look forward to and that brings you benefits if you follow these ideas. In the following chapter, we will concentrate on developing a healthy foundation by learning how to manage stress, getting enough sleep, and changing our perspective. You can build a solid foundation that will serve as a support system for you in all aspects of your life if you pay attention to all aspects of your health and well-being.

Chapter 4

WEEK 3 BUILD A HEALTHY BASIS BY MANAGING STRESS, GETTING ENOUGH SLEEP, AND CHANGING YOUR ATTITUDE

Hello, and welcome to the third week of the Body Reset! Managing stress, getting enough sleep, and maintaining a positive mindset will be the primary focuses of this week's activities.

But why exactly is it so crucial that you give your attention to these aspects of your health and well-being? Only a handful of the causes are as follows:

Management of stress: Prolonged exposure to stress can have a detrimental effect on both a person's physical and mental health. It can cause your immune system to become compromised, raise the likelihood that you will develop heart disease and other illnesses, and add to feelings of anxiety and despair in you. You can improve both your physical and mental well-being by becoming more skilled at stress management.

Sleep: Getting a sufficient amount of sleep is critical for one's overall health. During the time that you are asleep, your body works on repairing and regenerating itself, while your brain works on processing and consolidating memories. A lack of sleep has been linked to a range of negative health effects, such as the increased risk of heart disease, impaired immune function, and increased likelihood of weight gain. You may improve your overall health and well-being by making sleep a higher priority in your life.

Your frame of mind can have a significant influence on your physical and mental health, and vice versa. Your ability to deal with obstacles and failures, as well as your level of resiliency and tenacity, can all be improved by cultivating a more positive mental attitude. A pessimistic outlook, on the other hand, can prevent you from progressing toward your objectives and make it more difficult to do so. You can make improvements to your physical health and mental well-being simply by training your thoughts to be more optimistic.

How, then, can you establish a healthy foundation through the management of stress, the quality of your sleep, and your mindset? Try your hand at some of these different strategies:

You can manage your stress by **practicing stress management**

techniques such as deep breathing, meditation, and journaling, to name a few. There are many different techniques available for you to try. Try a variety of methods to determine which approach is most successful for you.

Make getting enough sleep a top priority. To enhance the quality of your sleep, you should strive to maintain a regular sleep schedule, develop a soothing bedtime routine, and ensure that your sleeping environment is comfortable. Stay away from electronic screens (such as phones and laptops) in an hour or so leading up to bedtime, as the blue light they emit can interfere with your natural sleep cycle. Caffeine and alcohol are both things that should be avoided close to bedtime because they might cause disruptions in sleep.

Cultivate a positive mindset: To cultivate a positive mindset, try to focus on the things that you are grateful for, practice positive affirmations, and surround yourself with positive people. This will help you cultivate a positive mindset. It would be best if you also made an effort to be nice to yourself and give yourself some leeway when things don't go the way you had intended.

Put healthy habits at the top of your to-do list. To put healthy habits at the top of your to-do list, try setting small goals that are within your reach and reward yourself when you achieve them. You can also keep track of your progress and praise yourself as you reach milestones.

Maintain an active lifestyle: To maintain an active lifestyle, you should seek out physical activities that you both enjoy and that are compatible with your lifestyle. This could include working out and playing sports, taking long walks, and tending a garden. Discovering activities that you look forward to performing is the most crucial thing there is to do.

Consume a varied and well-balanced diet: If you want to keep up a healthy diet, you should aim to eat a wide variety of whole and nourishing foods. This involves opting for meals that have been processed to a minimum, have a high nutrient content, and are enjoyable to consume. Steer clear of overly processed foods as well as those that include a lot of added sugar, salt, and fats that aren't good for you.

Maintain proper hydration: You should try to consume at least 8 cups (64 ounces) of fluids daily. The ideal option is water, but you can also acquire fluids from other sources, such as fruits, vegetables, and soups made with broth.

To successfully manage stress, you must first determine the factors contributing to it and then search for appropriate responses. This could be accomplished through techniques for managing stress, such as deep breathing, meditation, or exercise; it could also be accomplished through activities that help you relax, such as reading, writing, or spending time with friends and family; or it could be accomplished through a combination of these two approaches.

You may establish a healthy foundation in terms of managing stress, getting enough sleep, and maintaining a positive mindset by following these steps. This will assist you in reaching your health and fitness goals as well as feeling better overall.

After finishing the Body Reset, you may ensure that your health and well-being continue to improve by implementing these additional measures. Keep in mind that consistently maintaining your healthy routines and having patience with yourself are both extremely important. It takes time to build new habits and see success, but if you put in a little effort and commit yourself to the process, you can make long-lasting improvements in both your health and your well-being.

When you need assistance, it is essential to look for it. Feel free to seek assistance if you're finding it difficult to maintain your healthy habits or if you're experiencing feelings of being overwhelmed. You may seek help from people close to you, such as friends and family, or a medical professional.

On your successful completion of the Body Reset, congratulations! Only three weeks have passed since you started making significant changes to improve your health. You have learned how to nourish your body with whole, nourishing foods by following the simple strategies that are backed by science in this program. You have also learned how to boost your energy and metabolism by exercising and moving your body. Finally, you have learned how to create a healthy foundation by managing stress, getting enough sleep, and having a positive mindset.

Remember that the Body Reset is just the first step in the process. You must continue to lead a healthy lifestyle if you want to keep your current level of health and well-being. This includes consuming meals that nourish the body, remaining active, learning to manage stress, getting adequate sleep, and developing a happy mental attitude.

Last but not least, remember that it is acceptable to occasionally partake in sweets or deviate from the healthy routines you have established for yourself. It is essential to treat oneself kindly and to create a healthy balance that is appropriate for oneself. You can preserve your health and well-being throughout your life if you can strike a healthy balance and remain steadfast in your commitment to practicing healthy behaviors.

You may bring about a substantial improvement in both your health and well-being with only a little bit of work and dedication. Cheers to enjoying excellent health for the rest of your life! Another round of congratulations is for you on finishing the Body Reset and making such great journey in improving your health and well-being! Cheers to enjoying excellent health for the rest of your life!

Chapter 5

BRINGING IT ALL TOGETHER: HOW TO MAKE YOUR BODY RESET YOUR LIFESTYLE

You may be wondering how to incorporate more healthy routines and choices into your life now that you've finished the Body Reset program. This is a natural question to have at this point. The following are some suggestions that can help you bring everything together and turn the Body Reset into a lifestyle:

Beginning on a small scale is crucial because change can be unsettling; therefore, it is essential to begin on a small scale and make gradual modifications over time. This will allow you time to acclimate to the new routine and ensure that it becomes a habit.

Establish a balance: It is essential to locate a balance that is compatible with both your way of life and your preferences. This can entail giving in to the urge to eat something sweet once in a while or skipping a workout on a certain day. The essential thing is to strike a balance that enables you to take pleasure in life while still making decisions that are beneficial to your health.

Keep things straightforward, and don't try to make drastic changes to every aspect of your life at once.

Focus on making just one or two adjustments at a time and then build off that. You will be more likely to maintain your healthy routines if you keep things as straightforward as possible.

Find activities and routines that you want to do and that are appropriate for your lifestyle to make it more fun. This will increase the likelihood that you will continue practicing your healthy routines and incorporating them into your daily activities.

Feel free to ask for assistance if you're finding it difficult to maintain your healthy routines or if you're experiencing feelings of being overwhelmed. Seek support. You may seek help from people close to you, such as friends and family or a medical professional.

Maintain your motivation: Maintaining your motivation requires seeking sources of inspiration and encouragement. This could be accomplished through the use of support groups, personal accountability partners, or social media groups. You could also reward yourself for accomplishing goals that are within your reach and setting those goals.

Continue your education: If you want to continue making progress toward greater health and well-being, one of the most important things you can do is remain knowledgeable and up-to-date on the most recent studies and recommendations. You can accomplish this goal by reading articles, following reliable sources on social media, and having a conversation with a nutritionist or a healthcare expert.

Have a flexible mindset: if life gets in the way, it's good to depart from your healthy routine every once in a while. You must get back on course as soon as you can and do not allow a single obstacle to derail your progress.

You can make the body Reset a lifestyle by practicing these tips and remaining committed to your existing healthy habits. This will allow you to continue making progress toward improved health and wellness. Keep in mind that your trip is not a destination; you must maintain your healthy routines constantly and have patience with yourself. You can make more long-lasting changes in your health and well-being with a little effort and commitment.

Chapter 6

The following information is included in the "Bonus Tips and Techniques for Success section" of "The Body Reset: Rebuild Your Health in Only 3 Weeks with Easy, Science-Backed Strategies":

Make a plan: If you want to make eating healthily easier, attempt to develop a plan for the entire week. This may involve preparing meals and snacks in advance, as well as establishing a grocery list, packing lunches for work or school, and packing snacks for road trips. If you plan, you may assure that you will have time to prepare nutritious meals even when you are pressed for time.

Maintain a well-stocked pantry and refrigerator with healthy foods. One of the easiest ways to eat healthily is to maintain a well-stocked pantry and refrigerator with nutritious foods. This might consist of whole grains, legumes, nuts, seeds, fruits, vegetables, and proteins that are good for you. It is much simpler to prepare wholesome meals and snacks if you keep healthy goods in your pantry and refrigerator.

Have a flexible mindset, as it is acceptable to depart from your food plan on occasion or to enjoy a sweet treat now and again. The most important thing is to establish a healthy balance that works for you and to maintain your healthy routines consistently. Whenever you find yourself getting off track, try not to be too hard on yourself and get back on track as quickly as you possibly can.

It is important to avoid skipping meals because doing so can lead to later overeating and can make it more difficult to select healthy options. You should make an effort to eat meals and snacks at regular intervals to maintain a consistent level of energy and to keep your metabolism going.

Being hydrated is essential to preserving your health and well-being, so make sure to drink plenty of fluids throughout the day. Water should be your primary source of hydration, and you should strive to drink at least 8 cups' worth (64 ounces) of fluids every single day.

You can also obtain fluids from other sources, such as fresh fruits and vegetables as well as soups that are based on broth.

Maintain an active lifestyle: To maintain an active lifestyle, you should seek out physical activities that you both enjoy and that are compatible with your lifestyle. This could be everything from working out and playing sports to taking long walks and tending a garden. Discovering activities that you look forward to performing is the most crucial thing there is to do.

To successfully manage stress, you must first determine the factors that contribute to it and then search for appropriate responses to those factors. This could be accomplished through techniques for managing stress such as deep breathing, meditation, or exercise; it could also be accomplished through activities that help you relax, such as reading, writing, or spending time with friends and family; or it could be accomplished through a combination of these two approaches.

Don't be afraid to ask for assistance if you're finding it difficult to maintain your healthy routines or if you're experiencing feelings of being overwhelmed. Seek support. You may seek help from people close to you, such as friends and family, or a medical professional.

After you have finished the Body Reset, you can set yourself up for success and ensure that your health and well-being continue to improve if you follow these hints and suggestions. Keep in mind that consistently maintaining your healthy routines and having patience with yourself are both extremely important. It takes time to build new habits and to see success, but if you put in a little amount of effort and commit yourself to the process, you can make improvements that are long-lasting in both your health and your well-being.

Chapter 7

Consuming food that is good for you and well-balanced is an essential component of preserving your health and well-being. In this chapter, we have provided you with a recipe and a guide for meal planning to assist you in getting started.

All of the recipes included in this book have been created to be wholesome, delicious, and simple to put together. They contain complete components that have been processed only to a minimal extent and are abundant in nutrients including fiber, protein, and healthy fats.

We've included a weekly meal plan that gives you five different alternatives for breakfast, lunch, and supper each day to make organizing your meals easier. We have also provided you with a shopping list containing all the ingredients you will require for the upcoming week.

As you continue through the Body Reset, we suggest that you begin by following the meal plan and recipes provided for Week 1, and then go on to Weeks 2 and 3 as you move forward. You are more than welcome to combine different recipes and make any necessary adjustments to better fit your tastes and dietary requirements.

We have included recipes and a meal plan in this book to help you

support your health and well-being
by fueling your body with foods that
are whole and nourishing!

Week 1 Food Plan:

Monday:

Breakfast: Oatmeal with berries and almonds was prepared overnight and served for **breakfast.**

Lunch: Quinoa and black bean salad

Dinner: Chicken cooked on the grill served with roasted veggies.

Tuesday:

Toast topped with avocado and eggs: that'll be **breakfast.**

Wraps filled with turkey and spinach for **lunch**

Dinner: lentil soup made in a slow cooker

Wednesday:

Breakfast consists of a smoothie dish containing bananas, spinach, and chia seeds.

Salmon is prepared on the grill and served with quinoa and broccoli that has been cooked for **lunch**.

Sweet potato covered with black beans, salsa, and guacamole that have been baked and served as **dinner.**

Thursday:

Breakfast consists of Greek yogurt mixed with a variety of fruit and almonds.

Kale and quinoa salad with roasted veggies were for **lunch** today.

Tofu skewers on the grill with brown rice and steamed asparagus for **supper.**

Friday:

Scrambled eggs served with tomato slices and toast made with whole grain for **breakfast.**

Lunch: Hummus and veggie wrap

Dinner: turkey chili made in a slow cooker.

Saturday:

Breakfast consists of an omelet stuffed with vegetables and bread made with nutritious grains.

Skewers of grilled chicken and vegetables were served for **lunch.**

Spaghetti squash topped with marinara sauce and steamed broccoli constituted the **dinner.**

Sunday:

Pancakes made with whole grains served with yogurt and fruit for **breakfast.**

Brown rice and bean bowl topped with avocado and salsa as a healthy **lunch** option

Dinner: pork chops cooked on the grill, roasted sweet potatoes, and green beans cooked in water.

Shopping List:

Oats

Berries (such as strawberries, blueberries, or raspberries) (such as strawberries, blueberries, or raspberries)

Almonds

Quinoa

Beanzas Negras

Spinach

Avocado

Eggs

Bread made with whole grains

Turkey

Wraps made from whole grains

Lentils

Banana

Chia seeds (chia seeds)

Salmon

Broccoli

Sweet potatoes

Beanzas Negras

Salsa

Greek yogurt

Nuts (such as almonds or walnuts) (such as almonds or walnuts)

Kale

Tofu

Rice with a brown crust

Asparagus

Tomatoes

Hummus

Chapter 8

COMMONLY ASKED QUESTIONS WITH ANSWERS

In this chapter, we will provide answers to some of the questions that are asked the most frequently regarding the Body Reset program.

Is it risky to do the Body Reset?

A: The Body Reset is very safe for the vast majority of users. Despite this, it is always a good idea to speak with a healthcare professional before beginning any new diet or exercise program. This is especially important to do if you are currently taking medications or suffer from a medical condition.

If I have food sensitivities or allergies, is it possible for me to

continue with the Body Reset program?

A: If you suffer from food allergies or sensitivities, you need to select recipes and components that are appropriate for your dietary needs. You may need to make some alterations or adjustments to the recipes to make them work for you. You may also find it helpful to consult with a nutritionist or a healthcare practitioner for direction.

Can I still do the Body Reset even though I maintain a vegetarian or vegan diet?

A: Yes, The Body Reset cookbook has meals that may be followed by vegetarians as well as vegans. However, depending on your preferences and requirements, you might need to make some adjustments or alterations to the recipes. You may also find it helpful to consult with a nutritionist or a healthcare practitioner for direction.

A common question regarding the Body Reset is how long it will take to finish.

A: The Body Reset is intended to be finished in three weeks. On the other hand, you can go through the program as many times as you like and implement the ideas into your regular activities whenever you please.

If I am pregnant or nursing, is it safe for me to follow the Body Reset program?

A: In general, it is not advisable to maintain a restrictive diet when pregnant or breastfeeding, and the Body Reset is no exception to this rule. For the sake of both your health and your kid's health, it is essential to consume adequate nutrients. It is always a good idea to check with a healthcare practitioner before beginning any new diet or fitness program, especially if you are concerned about your health.

Will I experience weight loss when using the Body Reset?

A: The Body Reset is not particularly geared at achieving weight loss goals. Nonetheless, following the regimen may result in weight loss for certain individuals. Enhancing one's general health and sense of well-being is the program's primary goal.

If I have a medical issue, is it possible for me to still do the Body Reset?

A: Before beginning the Body Reset or any other new diet or fitness program, it is essential to discuss your medical history with a qualified medical expert, especially if you already have an existing health condition. They will be able to advise you on whether the program is safe for you to participate in and suggest any required alterations.

If I'm already taking medicine, is it safe for me to do the Body Reset?

A: Before beginning the Body Reset or any other new diet or fitness regimen, you must consult a medical practitioner if you are currently using any medication. Some medications can have an adverse reaction when combined with particular meals or nutrients; your healthcare provider will be able to provide you with any necessary changes.

If I am an athlete or lead a very busy lifestyle, is it possible for me to continue with the Body Reset program?

A: The Body Reset is perfectly safe for the vast majority of individuals, even active people like athletes and those who live an active lifestyle. However, before beginning any new diet or exercise program, speaking with a healthcare professional or sports nutritionist is always a good idea. This is especially important to do if you have specific requirements or objectives.

If I am beyond the age of 50, can I continue with the Body Reset program?

A: Indeed, The Body Reset is completely risk-free for the vast majority of people, including those who are beyond the age of 50. But, before beginning any new diet or fitness regimen, it is always a good idea to check with a healthcare practitioner, particularly if you have any health problems or are currently taking drugs.

If I am less than 18 years old, can I still participate in the body Reset?

A: Indeed, the Body Reset is perfectly safe for the vast majority of people, including those who are less than 18 years old. However, before beginning any new diet or exercise program, speaking with a healthcare professional or parent is always a good idea, particularly if you have any health concerns or are still growing and developing. This is especially important for younger people.

We hope that some of your inquiries regarding the Body Reset program have been addressed by this chapter. If you have any more inquiries, please do not be reluctant to consult with a nutritionist or a healthcare professional for further direction.

Conclusion

Honoring Your Struggles and Triumphs Along the Path to Health and Well-being.

On your successful completion of the Body Reset, congratulations! We hope that you have gained some useful techniques for enhancing your health and well-being and that you now feel empowered to make some long-term changes in your life as a result of the information that you have obtained here.

The path to improved health and wellness is not always simple, but it is unquestionably worthwhile. You can significantly improve your health and well-being by bringing about gradual shifts in the routines and attitudes you follow on a day-to-day basis.

We want to encourage you to continue making healthy living a part of your lifestyle by applying the ideas you learned from the Body

Reset to your daily routine. Keep in mind that consistently maintaining your healthy routines and having patience with yourself are both extremely important. It takes time to build new habits and to see success, but if you put in a little amount of effort and commit yourself to the process, you can make improvements that are long-lasting in both your health and your well-being.

Take some time to celebrate your accomplishments and the progress you've made while you think back on your journey through the Body Reset program. As you do this, you'll be able to see how far you've come. You must acknowledge and appreciate your hard work, regardless of whether you have decreased your body fat percentage, increased your energy levels, or improved your overall health and well-being.

Spend some time reflecting on how far you've come on your path to health and well-being, and don't be afraid to talk to others about what you've learned along the way. You never know who you might motivate to make positive changes in their own lives; perhaps it will be someone else.

Creating brand-new objectives for yourself is a good approach to recognizing and appreciating the progress you've made. This may have anything to do with your physical health, like getting in shape for a race or building up your stamina and strength. It's also possible that it has anything to do with your overall health and wellness, like relieving stress or making your mental health better.

One further technique to commemorate your achievements is to give yourself a reward that you take pleasure in doing. This may be something simple, such as a massage or a new workout clothing, or it could be something more involved, such as a trip or a memorable meal. The most essential thing is to make sure that you give yourself some recognition and rewards for all of the hard work that you have done.

And finally, don't be embarrassed to tell others about your accomplishments and the lessons you've learned. You never know who you might motivate to make positive changes in their own lives; perhaps it will be someone else. Sharing your experience can also give you a sense of accountability, keeping you motivated and on track as you progress with your goals.

We hope that you have found the Body Reset program to be a helpful resource and that you are pleased with the progress that you have achieved as a result of using the program. Keep in mind that the process of improving your health and wellness is an ongoing one; therefore, you must maintain your healthy habits and continue to engage in decision-making that is beneficial to your well-being. Cheers to the continuation of your good health and well-being!

Pharm. Charity O., is a highly knowledgeable and experienced healthcare professional with a passion for assisting others in achieving optimal health and wellness. Pharm. Charity has extensive knowledge of the most recent findings in scientific research and a solid foundation in the field of pharmacology. She offers a straightforward strategy that is supported by data for altering your health in as little as three weeks. The strategies that are outlined in this book are designed to be straightforward, doable, and extremely efficient. As a result, it will be easy for readers to implement these strategies into their day-to-day lives.